Pilates

Step-by-step Instruction Exercises to Improve Pilates Exercises

(Core Pilates Exercises and Easy Sequences to Practice at Home)

Peter Rodriguez

Published By **Tyson Maxwell**

Peter Rodriguez

All Rights Reserved

Pilates: Step-by-step Instruction Exercises to Improve Pilates Exercises (Core Pilates Exercises and Easy Sequences to Practice at Home)

ISBN   978-1-9995502-3-3

Legal & Disclaimer

The information contained in this book is not designed to replace or take the place of any form of medicine or professional medical advice. The information in this book has been provided for educational & entertainment purposes only.

The information contained in this book has been compiled from sources deemed reliable, and it is accurate to the best of the Author's knowledge; however, the Author cannot guarantee its accuracy and validity and cannot be held liable for any errors or omissions. Changes are periodically made to this book. You must consult your doctor or get professional medical advice before using any of the suggested remedies, techniques, or information in this book.

Table Of Contents

Chapter 1: What Is Classical Pilates?

Pilates is a set of exercises controlled by a trainer that aim at building the strength of your base (Powerhouse) as well as strengthen alignment and posture as well as improve the flexibility of the spine and joints. Pilates is fitness for the whole body and was created in the early days of Joseph Pilates. The combination of breathing exercises that are controlled allows Pilates not just an exercise for the body but can also help in focusing your mind by establishing a link between mind and body. When we speak of Classical Pilates we are talking about the old-fashioned method of training. Joseph Pilates created the exercises that are not the same as Pilates which is taught in the classroom (think of the term "classical" in the world of classical music). While Classical Pilates does often take form in a class or a studio. Classical Pilates has a set exercise routine for beginners to intermediate, advanced as well as advanced level. This book is only focusing on beginner exercises. Joseph Pilates created this set sequence of exercises as Pilates believed that these exercises complement one another and counter-extended one another, which meant that it would result in an overall balanced workout that will yield the most effective results.

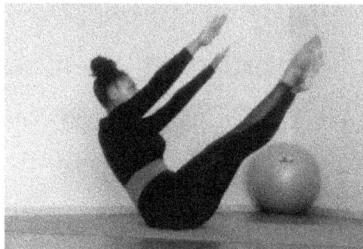

Joseph Pilates

Joseph Pilates was born in 1883 in Germany. He was the son of a professional gymnast which sparked his love for movement. Joseph suffered from frequent illness and he made the decision to be a bodybuilder and gymnast as his father did and devoted all of his life to improving his fitness and health. In this period, he came to an idea that poor posture, bad breathing, and stress from everyday routines were responsible for poor mental and physical well-being. In this light, the doctor devised a sequence of exercises. Joseph relocated to England and earned a decent living by being a fighter and self-defence instructor at several police schools. Then, during World War 1 Joseph got detained by British authorities. During his confinement, he instructed the other internees. In this is when he truly improved his training using the equipment that was available in the confines of his prison, and was able to call his work as contrology. Once he was released, after his release, he went to Germany to work with specialists in the field of physical health as well as dancing. Then he moved towards his home in the United States. When he arrived in the States He met his wife Clara and they established the first Pilates Studio in NYC. Through the cooperation with dance instructors, the majority of his students were ballet dancers. Joseph was constantly improving his techniques. Additionally, he was influenced by the movements of animals.

In the light of all that, Pilates developed his Classical Pilates exercises that we have today and are able to master through this guide. In the midst of his 83 years, Joseph Pilates past away in New York (in 1967).

Powerhouse

The Powerhouse in the first chapter. However, what exactly does it mean?

Powerhouse in Classical Pilates means: Powerhouse is a reference to Classical Pilates means:

The abdominal muscles are the most commonly affected (4 layers)

1.Transversus abdominis (deepest layer)

2. Internal Obliques (side abdominals, 2nd layer)

3. External Obliques (side abdominals 3rd layer)

4.Rectus abdominis (outer layer six pack)

The thighs' inner parts

- The muscles of the butt

All working as one strong group.

The majority of exercises taught that are performed in Classical Pilates are initiated from the Powerhouse (predominantly the abdominal muscles) which is to help strengthen the Powerhouse. Joseph Pilates believed that all right movements start in the Powerhouse which is why his belief was that a healthy Powerhouse ensures the longevity of your body.

The six Pilates fundamentals

Joseph Pilates created all his exercises using just six

The principles that you have in your minds.

* Concentration

* Control

* Centering

* Precision

* Breathing

* Flow

Concentration

The information you'll find in this guide, Classical Pilates exercises and transitions from one activity to the next are extremely particular. Concentration is among the fundamental principles of pilates to get optimal results for any exercise that you take part in. Concentration may sound like a simple concept, yet in my personal experience, there are times when I'm working but I'm distracted by another thing. When I do this, I am not focused on the job that I'm doing, and it shows up in the final results. Sometimes, the results aren't so good those when I'm focused. It is the same for doing Classical Pilates. As you continue to practice focus and concentration, the better become at it, and the greater the benefits from your Pilates training will be. This is not only on a physical but also the mental side.

Control

If we do Pilates there are a variety of things come together.

There are many things to be considered:

Our breath

How our limbs and tendons are up to

- engaging our Powerhouse

the movement that actually takes place during the exercise

Coordination

Listening to corrections and synchronization

In order to perform exercises to the highest possible level, in addition to being focused, we must have control over the body's movements to link the various elements of our body together. This also is a result of practice and getting familiar with the workouts.

Centering

Like we have already discussed, every one of the Classical Pilates exercises are initiated by the Powerhouse at the heart of our body. It begins with slowing down your mind (concentration) and body. While we are lying on the mat prior to when we begin our workouts We want to be sure that we're in a good place upon the mat. The limbs we work on are equal distance away from the centerline. Also, we begin our workouts at a distance from the centreline. Then, when we progress and get more the control we will be able to move far away from centreline. (Example legs that are hundreds of inches long The more advanced the lower the legs are, they move further away from the center in the human body.)

Precision

Precision is a result of focus and discipline. Our focus and control to complete exercises to the highest accuracy of our abilities. The practice of Classical Pilates we are very particular about how many times we repeat every exercise since we concentrate more on the performance of our exercises rather than amount of repetitions. We are trying to make sure that our body isn't tired and start compensating for other joints and muscles which is not the intention of the workout. It is important to perform exercises with maximum ability, while engaging the Powerhouse to get the most effective outcomes. This is why precision is among the six fundamentals of Classical Pilates.

Breathing

Joseph Pilates believed that poor breathing was among the causes of unhealthy well-being. Breathing is essential to ensure blood circulation and for cells within the body to function efficiently. Inhaling can help to engage the abdominal muscles and create an interaction between the your body and your mind. Breathing in Classical Pilates exercises also creates movement through the exercises. When we practice Pilates we mostly use the higher ribs and back breathing instead of breathing through the lower abdomen so that we remain as abdominal muscles contracted to the maximum extent possible, and create a strong powerhouse to perform each exercise out of. In general, we inhale when we are in the extension position and exhale during the flexion (contraction) and turning (rotation). Examples: during the exercise Spine stretching forward, we inhale while sitting in a straight position (extension) and exhale as we extend our arms forward to above (flexion).

Flow

While Pilates is all about the control and precision, we seek to achieve fluidity through the use of the breath in conjunction with the exercise. Pilates is meant to be an exercise with the principles the above mentioned principles to be in the mind. When we are able to establish the exercises and the five principles, we must integrate the movement. From exercise to exercise in an appropriate transition, making your Pilates exercise a continuous practice that should be continued until you are able to complete the Push Up series towards the end. That's what we strive toward. However, if you're working alongside novices, you may need occasionally stop for in order to talk about or explain the concept, especially if you're looking to get closer on some exercises. The more advanced you are, the more fluid the exercise is likely to be. However, I would like to point out that even when you're teaching beginners, you will need to create something that flows in your practice and the class is still going to be a fitness session. This can be difficult for instructors initially, but once they have the proper training and practice, it'll become more comfortable.

Chapter 2: Learn In A Secure Environment

Be sure to ensure that before you are ready to teach, your space is well-organized, both in order to protect your health that also look professional for an instructor. Check the temperature in the classroom. Be sure that it's not warm or cold. If you're in a place you're unfamiliar with, be sure you're aware of you can go in case of emergency.

You can teach the basics using your Powerhouse

In your role as an Pilates instructor, it's crucial that you instruct by using your Powerhouse. That means that from the time students enter the room and during the time that you teach your class until they exit your class, you'll be a model for them, showing good posture. It is not possible to tell them to "straighten your back long" to your pupils when yourself have a an incline.

Use your voice

In addition to teaching from the comfort of your Powerhouse You should be aware of your voice. Since your Classical Pilates class is mainly spoken, take note of the volume and the dynamics that your voice produces. Your goal is to provide your students a challenge, however you must also create a fun environment so that they'll want to come back. It is possible to increase the volume and the dynamic, or rhythm of your voice if you are trying to inspire your students during a tough workout. You can also calm your vocal tone a little as you begin and finish your class. Be sure that your students be able to hear you clearly so that they can know what's going on or the topic to concentrate on.

Correcting errors

While teaching, you'll provide corrections to your students. Make sure to give at least 2 or 3 corrections verbally for each exercise! This will help your students to complete the task with as much precision as they can. There are 3 methods to guide your students.

- Verbally

Touch

- By demonstrating

- Verbally

In the event that you have to correct verbally your students, I'd recommend that you rectify in a positive manner. What I mean is to verbally state your goals for what you wish to encourage or want to encourage, instead of stating what you would not like your children to take part in.

As an example, instead of declaring "don't arch your lower back in the hundreds".

The way to describe it is: "pull your abs towards your spine to plant the lower back into the mat".

This means that you're instructing your students in be in the right posture for the exercises.

Touch

Touch

If you are using contact to help your students learn it is important to be aware as an educator. As not everybody likes being at all. If you decide to touch someone to correct them, you could contact them, or slowly move your fingers. A gradual touch refer to starting with a gentle contact to inform them to rectify them, and then applying some pressure slowly. It is essential to be mindful of the quality of the touch. Nothing is more unpleasant than a feel that's as if it was a tickle or touch that's too hard. Make sure to use good sense when you use touches. If you do decide to make contact with someone, you must be aware of the goal you want to accomplish with your gesture. If you are unsure, don't contact them and instead make a verbal correction or even a display.

- Demonstration

We have discussed previously that Classical Pilates is taught verbally. This is so that students are able to work according to their abilities rather than trying to emulate the teacher's instructions and impose on their themselves into the exercises which could cause injury to themselves. Pilates is a method that you must practice, and the more you do it the better you'll get. However, there will be times in your class when you are able to show some exercises or demonstrate the accuracy or prudence of the exercise. We try to make it as minimally as we can.

Use of words with a sense of humour

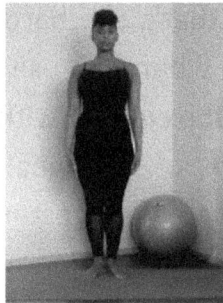

Like we've discussed previously, Classical Pilates is mainly instructed verbally. As Classical Pilates is meant to be a fitness class, we'd want to ensure that the flow is maintained within the class. One way to do this is to be clever with the words you speak.

Be as brief and precise as possible in your sentences. Examples: For instance, instead of using the phrase "And now we are going to bend our knees in the chest to set up for the Hundreds". It could be "Bend knees in chest for the Hundreds". Look for shortcuts to help your students get in the direction you would like them to go in order to are able to more easily improve them, and concentrate on precision and flow. This will take some time to master at first. However, I'd like to encourage you to take an initial class with your friends or relatives to learn this important technique. It will make a huge distinction in the way you become a successful Classical Pilates teacher.

Fun teacher

The exercises and structure of Classical Pilates are very specific which can result in the classes quite strict. While you'd like keep to your prescribed schedule and the format, you'll would like to make your class engaging and enjoyable so students will want to return. Be prepared and let your students put in the effort and also enjoy a more. Use jokes or imaginative phrases to encourage your students into an appropriate position. Example: Instead of using the phrase "Squeeze your butt muscles". The alternative is to say "hold on to a $100 with butt". Students will continue to work their butt muscles, however it will give the exercise ease and enjoyment.

Keep in mind that we all experience bad days at times, However, when you teach an class, I want to remind students to remember that you're there for the benefit of your students. Your job is to inspire students and teach your students something new and exciting. Be sure to keep your bad day in the class. Students will be down also. Be aware to the energetic of your students and make adjustments according to their needs. Talk to your students following the class, and be always encouraging and inspiring.

Stance, teacher posture and warm-up exercises

Pilates Stance

Before we begin our exercise it is important to ensure we have a well-aligned location to be working starting. For Classical Pilates we call that posture Pilates Stance.

Let's look at the Pilates posture starting from the bottom and ending at the top.

Feet are placed in a V-position The toes are placed 2 feet wide apart.

heels meet.

They are also straight and the knees have not been too stretched, or

The knees bend and the knees are pulled upwards towards the thighs

The thighs are in contact and rotate in the direction of the sides.

* The muscles in the butt region are squeezed to form a tight band.

* The abs are pulled back towards the spine.

19

The back of the car is straight.

In the ribs, the ribs get pulled into

* The arms sit beside the body. The shoulders are

Down pulled into the shoulder blades

The shoulders of both are at the same level.

The chest is large and wide

Neck length is lengthy

* Chin runs in line with the floor. it is possible to make a fist with it.

Chest and chin

* Gaze is in the direction of forward

* The head's top extends to the ceiling

This is the best assessment of the Pilates posture. You will notice that your students have diverse positions. Perhaps you have one of your students with knee injuries. They won't have the ability to keep their heels in a Pilates position. This is why you need to should ensure that the student is able to perform the exercise within their capabilities. Teachers need to recognize these poses, and also be aware to not push students into positions they're not able to perform anatomically. That's why it's crucial to learn and remember specific postures, and also to conduct an internal study of human anatomy.

Teachers pose

It is crucial as teachers to model using your Powerhouse and to be aware of the posture you take while giving lessons. The Pilates position is the foundation for the posture your instructor will use. It is the posture you will use in the class when teaching. Do you walk around while your abs are pulled tight? Are you sitting on your knees with a slack back? The best way to assess the posture of your body by following the principles of a perfect Pilates posture on preceding pages. It is not a requirement that you should move your feet in a straight line constantly, however, it can be helpful to look at your posture to determine where and what you can do to improve the posture of your teacher. By doing this, you'll provide a good model and example to your pupils.

Chapter 3: Exercises For Warming Up

Prior to starting the complete Classical Pilates beginners order, you can choose to complete 2-3 warm up exercises. If you're able to spare the time to spare, you may decide to perform just one or two exercises at the end of class. The warm-up exercises are snippets of some of the complete Classical Pilates exercises. Your students know certain postures. This is why the aim of the warm-up exercises is not only to warm your body, but also to improve and practice several of the essential components of the Classical Pilates order. Like how to work your abs and hold the ribs tight while lifting your arms close to your ears. Here we will look at a few ideas of exercises are suitable for you to try. It's perfectly acceptable to incorporate your own warm-up exercises however, make sure they're not only there to help warm your pupil, but the exercises serve an ulterior motive, which are designed to complement and enhance your exercises within the Classical Pilates order.

Warm up exercises for standing

Certain of these exercises are able to do before beginning your hundreds, or even at the close of class. In every exercise the exact time of the program I'd recommend you to perform the exercises. If you want more information on the Classical Pilates journey find all the warm-up exercises listed found on the Classical Pilates Youtube Channel.

https://bit.ly/2Xhsybu

Head rolls

- Begin in Pilates posture and then roll your head towards the right side or

5 times before repeating five times, then repeat to the left

The head moves independently of the other parts of the body

Maintain the abs in a downward direction towards your spine.

Perform this workout before you get started on your entire training

Goals: Warming the neck

Shoulder rolls

Begin in Pilates posture and then roll your shoulder forward to 4 or 5

repeatedly, and repeat until the in the front

The shoulders move independently from the rest of the body

Maintain the abs in a downward direction towards your spine.

Perform this move prior to starting the complete exercise

Goals: Warming the shoulders and warming up the upper back.

Arm isolation

Begin in Pilates posture, bringing the arms to the

Ceiling next to ears, and finally reach towards the sides.

Repeat this 4 to 5 times

Maintaining the ribs tucked into

Keep abs tight

Moving the arms away from the rest of your body

Do this before beginning the entire training

Objectives: Warm the shoulders, master how to move your arms separately from the the body. Work on lifting the arms with the intention of not putting the ribs.

Standing cat & cow

Start by putting your legs slightly larger than the hips. The legs

Parallel

The knees should be bent slightly.

The spine should be rounded backwards Look into the your belly button

You can then arch your spine forward, gaze up towards the ceiling

Repeat this the process 4 to 5 times

Maintain the abs active

- Shoulders up

Use your breath

Perform this workout before you begin your full workout or when you are at

at the conclusion of the class

Goals: Warming up your spine and ribs, increasing the spinal flexibility

Hip isolation

Start by putting your legs slightly wider than your hips. Legs

Parallel

The knees should be bent slightly.

The pelvis is lifted both forward and back, as well as moving the pelvis side-to-side

- Repeat this 4-8 times

The hips should be moved apart from the rest body

Maintaining the abs in a state of engagement

Perform this workout before beginning the entire training or after

at the conclusion of the class

Goals: Warming the lower back and warming the hips, increasing flexibility both in the lower back and hips

Hip circle

Begin with legs slightly larger than the hips. The legs

Parallel

By bending the knees slightly, you can bend your knees

The hips should be rotated up to five times. after that, circle the hips

opposite direction

Moving the hips apart from the rest body

Keep the abs active

Perform this workout prior to beginning the entire training or after

The class is over at the end

Goals: Warming up lower back and warming the hips, and increasing flexibility within the lower back, and hips

Roll down

Begin in Pilates position

Arms extended towards the ceiling

- Spine that is articulate to the bottom and then back up

3 to 4 times

If hamstrings are tight, extend the legs while rolling

down

Maintain the abs engaged

The pelvis should remain still for as long as you can while rolling down

Perform this workout prior to starting the complete training or after

The class is over at the end

Objectives: Warming up your back, flexing the spine Learn how to

Flex the spine, stretch the hamstrings stretch

Parallel squats and then extended

Begin with legs slightly larger than the hips. Legs

Parallel or a little wider was later redesigned to be

Bend the legs, keeping the back straight

as possible

Repeat the process 4 to 6 times

If you bend your legs, the thighs will be aligned

until the level

Keep the abs active

- - Squeeze the butt muscles while straightening your legs

Do this prior to beginning the entire exercise or during

The class is over at the end

Goals: Warming up legs, strengthening the legs and

butt muscles

Ballet plie (Ballet squats)

Begin the exercise with the Ballet first posture (check

terminology list)

Hands in waist

The legs should be bent half in a straight back

(heels on the flooring) and bend your knees to the floor until you are able to bend

Lifting the heels a bit then come back down

- Repeat this 4 to 6 times

The moment you bend your legs to the fullest, keep your your heels to the

Floor

The more you lower is determined by how straight you're able to

Maintain your spine and aim to maintain your back as straight as you can.

as possible

Do this before that you get into the full training or after

at the conclusion of the class

Goals: Warming the legs, enhancing the legs, and

butt muscles

Arch with force

Start from the same position in a horizontal direction, in the middle or hip width or someplace in between

Start in Pilates position

Lift the heels up and take the ball of your foot one step at a

One or both of them simultaneously

Repeat the process 4-8 times

Maintaining your upper body as straight as you can.

Maintaining the abs in a state of engagement

Maintaining the muscles of the buttocks active

- Perform this exercise prior to you begin your full workout or after

The class is over at the end

Goals: Warming the feet, strengthening the legs as well as the butt muscles, calfs and calfs and balance exercises

Balance exercises

Start with parallel feet or with Pilates position

Then lift one leg upwards with the opposite leg straight on the floor.

on the floor, or to the heel of your feet for a greater level of

Keep the balance in place for 10 seconds

When you have held for 10 repetitions, you may turn to the left

After that, left and up after that back down

Do this before that you get into the full training or after

at the conclusion of the class

Abs Strengthening Goals: Strengthening abs helps increase focus and

Control

Warm up exercises for supine and sitting exercises

The majority of the exercises I do before the hundreds. However, there are a few other exercises that are not. Take a closer examine these tasks.

Baby Roll Back

Start from a sitting standing position. Bend your knees and the feet

Parallel flat mat on the mat

Be sure to hold onto your legs

and then roll the arms back, straightening the arms to make sure they are touching

place the lower part of the mat. Then, roll back to the mat.

Keep your abs in place

- Repeat the process 4 times

Make sure that the spine is in a C-curve whenever you return to the top,

Straighten your back in the final second

Be sure to look in the stomach

Perform this workout prior to starting the complete training

Goals: Engaging the lower abdominals, strengthening the abs in the lower part and warming the entire body, and practicing keeping your lower back in a curve

Baby roll back and flat and then back

Begin in a sitting in a seated position, knees bent and the feet

Parallel flat mat on the mat

Hold your legs back straight and look in the direction of

And then roll your eyes back into the stomach, and then straighten the arms

Try to place the lower back of the mat. Roll

return to straight line and then look back

Maintaining abs tight

Repeat the process four times

Maintain the spine in a C-curve in case you want to roll back up

Always keep an eye on the abdomen

- Perform this exercise prior to when you begin your full exercise

Goals: Engaging the lower abs, energizing the abs in the lower part while warming up the entire body, and practicing the differences

Between straight back and a C curvature

Arm isolation

Begin by supining by bending your knees and feet

Parallel flat mat on the mat

Reaching arms towards the ceiling, and after that raising arms

just behind the ear.

- Repeat this 4 to 6 times

The ribs should be tight

Maintain the abs active

- Hold your lower back on the mat

The shoulders are pulled to the back

Do this prior to starting the complete exercise

Objectives: Warming shoulders, gaining confidence to move your arms without affecting the other parts of the body, getting with arms right next to ears without burning the ribs.

Table top arm isolations

Start by putting yourself from a supine posture where the knees are bent at a 90o

angles, legs together place the toes in a in a parallel

Arms reaching to the ceiling and then lifting the arms

right next to the ear

Repeat the process the process 4 to 6 times

Make sure that the ribs are tight

Maintain the abs active

- Hold your lower back on the mat

The shoulders are pulled to the back

Do this before beginning the entire exercise

Objectives: Warming shoulders, learning to move your arms without affecting the remainder of the body. getting your arms close to the ears, without causing any discomfort to the ribs, triggering the abs in the lower part of the body, and learning to hold the lower rear in the mat

Dead bug

- Begin by supining in a position, by bending your knees to a 90o

angles, legs aligned and point toes in a towards each other

Arms reaching to the ceiling

Next, reach your right hand next to your an ear, and pull it back.

Left leg simultaneously return, and do it again.

the opposite leg and arm

- Repeat the process 4 to 6 times

Make sure that the ribs are kept in

Engage your abs

- Place the lower back of the mat

Shoulder muscles are pulled into the back

Perform this workout before you begin your full exercise

Goals: Warming the shoulders, understanding how to move arms without affecting the the body. Developing the ability to move the arms up to the ears, without damaging the ribs. working the lower abdominals and making sure to keep your lower back within the mat to enhance coordination

Chapter 4: Hip Isolations

Begin from a supine posture by bending your knees and feet

Parallel flat mat on the mat

Hip width is spaced at the hips

- Bringing the hips towards the ceiling, and then bending the back

- Repeat the process 4 to 6 times

Maintaining the abs in a state of engagement

The hips are moved in an isolation with the entire body

Do this before beginning the entire exercise or

prior to shoulder bridge

Goals: Warming up your lower back and increasing flexibility of the pelvis and lower back.

Table top taps that alternate.

Start by putting yourself from a supine posture where the knees are bent at an angle of 90o

angles, legs together make sure the toes are towards each other

Arms lie flat on the mat and are pointing away toward the

toes

- Tap your right foot on the mat, then lift it the toe back and repeat.

with left leg

- Repeat the process 4 to 6 times

Maintaining your lower back on the mat

Maintaining the abs in a state of engagement

Maintaining the ribs

- Perform this exercise prior to when you begin your full workout

Goals: Warming the lower abdominals, enhancing the abs lower, gaining knowledge how to keep the ribs and abs tight and

ensuring that the lower back stays in the mat

Double taps for table tops

Begin by supine, by bending your knees to a 90o

Angle, legs joined, make sure the toes are towards each other

The arms are placed flat on the mat, extending toward the

toes

Tap both feet onto the mat

Repeat this 4 to 6 times

Keep your lower back on the mat

Maintaining the abs in a state of engagement

Maintaining the ribs

Perform this workout prior to starting the complete training

Goals: Warming the lower abdominals, strengthening the lower abs, and learning how to keep abs and ribs engaged while maintaining your lower back within the mat

The shoulder and head lift

Begin by supine, using knees bent and feet

Flat and parallel on the mat

Arms extended to the ceiling

Head and shoulders from the mat between

The arms, lower shoulder and head are back the back of your shoulders and arms.

The mat

1. Lift your the head and shoulders, then extend arms

behind the ear to the ceiling and then the lower part of the head, and

shoulders back onto the mat

Variation 2: Moving arms in the direction of ears, lift the head

and then spread the shoulders out on and lay on the mat with the arms in the same direction as the mat.

ears and the lower and upper head as well as shoulders back into the mat

Repeat this 4 to 8 times

- - Look to the stomach when lifting the shoulders and the head.

Pull the abdominals into

- Lower back into the mat

Do this prior to starting the complete exercise

Objectives: Strengthening upper abdominals while warming up abs and the entire body.

Cat and cow

"Come on all fours!"

Turning the spine toward the ceiling, looking into the

Belly

- After that, he arched his back, looking up at the ceiling

Repeat this 4 to 8 times

Maintain the abs active

Perform this exercise immediately after or before your resting position or

Before the push up series

Goals: Warming up your spine and ribs. It also creates an increase in flexibility of the spine

Dead bug that has reversed

- Begin with all fours

- Straightening the right leg and arm simultaneously,

Leg is parallel and pointed

Repeat the opposite side and leg

Repeat this 4 - 6 times

Maintaining the abs in a state of engagement

In the reverse direction

Maintaining the straight back

Do this exercise immediately after or prior to resting place

Goals: Improve balance, improve focus, strengthen abs, lengthening spine

7. The complete order of Classical Pilates mat beginners exercises

In this section, we'll take a look at exercises on the Classical Pilates Mat beginners

exercises. On the next page, you will see a diagram that lists every exercise listed, along with the suggested repetitions, and a few additional notes. In this chapter, we'll go over each exercise thoroughly. Each exercise is described in the instructional videos that which are available at YouTube. YouTube Channel Classical Pilates. The Classical Pilates channel is the best. YouTube Channel you can also get a YouTube video showing the complete sequence of the exercises for beginners.

Hundreds

Repetitions: 100

* Inhale 5 pump and exhale 5 pumps 10 times (100)

Goals:

* Increases blood circulation

* Warming up of the body

* Strengthens abdominal muscles.

* Extends the length of the entire body

The setup:

* Chest knees in the chest.

* Lift your head and shoulder from the mat.

* Arms are lifted

* Turn your attention to the belly button

* Increase the length of the legs by in 45 degrees from the floor.

Beginner legs are straight up to at least the floor (proximal)

The lower the leg, more advanced (distal)

The legs should be at eye level (Really advanced)

* Point of pilates in feet (feet in V) heels placed together

Toes separated (point toes)

Set exercise in motion:

Start to pump your arms.

* Breathe in 2,3,4,5

* Breathe out 2,3,4,5

Corrections:

* Check the belly button

* Continue to lift shoulders off the mat.

Make sure to keep the lower back of your child firmly to the mat

* Make sure heels are kept together

* squeeze at the bottom (when legs stretch to 45

degrees)

Continue pulling your abs toward the spine.

* Remembering to breathe exhale 5 pumps inhale 5 pumps

Make sure to keep the head as well as the upper and lower body at a safe distance

Chapter 5: Pumping Up The Arms

Notes:

The way that your legs are able to be really based on whether you're able to keep the lower back firmly within the mat. This can be achieved through pulling your abs back by gluing your abs to the spine. Beginners should aim to raise your legs towards the ceiling while working in the proximal. As they advance, the further down the legs fall in working distal. The ideal position for the legs is at to eye level. Be sure to elevate knees with your chest first, before lifting your head from mat particularly for novices.

The transition from Roll-up to Transition:

* Knees and chest to the knees.

* Bring the head and shoulders into the mat.

* Reposition the arms into the mat.

Roll up

Repetitions:

* 5 times

Goals:

* The spine is articulated.

* Improve flexibility of the spine

* Stretching and lengthening the spine.

* Warm up of the spine and back.

* Strengthening abdominal muscles

The setup:

* Stand straight with your legs onto the mat

* Feet that are parallel and flexed.

* Legs joined (Legs could be hips with the legs separated) to

For beginners, it's best to put legs joined)

* Arms reach toward the ceiling

Set exercise in motion:

Inhale in the chin toward the chest. Then, slowly roll through the arms

* Maintain spine in C curvature, extend ahead and breathe in

* Pull abs deeper in

* Breathe in and then move your spine, and then return to the mat.

* Now reaching the arms to the ears, breathe in.

Corrections:

• Keep your heels moving away from the mat and keep pushing heels into the mat (when they are moving up)

* Shoulder stays to the side to the back

Maintain abs pulled toward the spine.

* Remain in the C curve while going up or down

* Continue lifting the ribs away from the hips as you reach to the side and up over

You can imagine playing with and over

*This isn't an hamstring stretch, but rather it is a stretch of the spine

* As you bring the arms to return them towards the ear your ribs

down

The transition to one leg circle

* Arms placed next to the body mat

One leg circle

Repetitions:

* 5 times each direction

Goals:

* Strengthen your legs

* Oil the hip joint

* Helps increase flexibility of the hips

The setup:

* Right knee injured in chest

* Place left leg on the mat with feet parallel to each other, and keep feet flexed

Straighten left leg until the ceiling

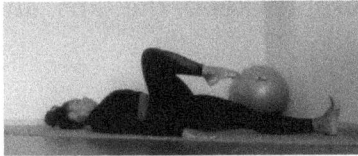

* Leg is turned inwards and foot directed

Make the exercise move:

* Breathe in and move right leg to left leg.

* Breathe in circle and back until you can walk straight

After 5 repetitions, reverse the circle.

* and switch leg

Corrections:

* Keep your foot on the mat in a seated position with the foot in a flexed position

* Make sure to keep the leg that is working straight with straight feet and straight legs.

The legs are pointed as you circle them

* Make sure to keep the abs and the ribs pulled tight

* Draw an outline of the ceiling using your feet

Then, focus on the ceiling.

* Make sure to keep your upper body and hips as straight as you can.

* Place your triceps on the mat in order to help to stabilize

The transition to Rolling as a ball

- Beginners

* Bring both knees to the chest.

* Grab hold of your thighs, and then the body up until sitting

the position

- Advanced beginner

Straighten both legs and place them on the mat and flex the feet

* Arms reaching toward the ceiling

* and then roll up until you are seated (Like the roll up

exercise)

The ball rolls like a roll

Repetitions:

* 8 times

Goals:

* Massaging de spine

Massage the pressure point on the spine

* Strengthening the abs

* Helps to control the body

Setting up:

Place your hands next to the buttocks. Lift yourself up

Forwards on mats

* Secure the ankles' outsides

* Lifting feet from the mat, feet to Pilates the point (heels

Toes apart)

* Knees to shoulders (Knees are not joined, however

Heels are in the same place)

* Forming a C-curve of the spine

* Looking at the belly button

* balancing your buttocks as if you were a ball

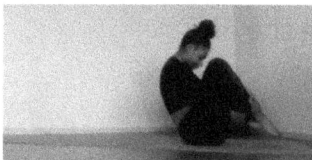

Make the exercise move:

Breathe deeply and breathe out and roll to the back

* Breathe deeply to breathe out and come again and regain your balance.

• Keep your feet away off the mat and pull the abs to

Corrections:

* Roll over shoulders. Neck and head aren't

pressing the mat while rolling to the back !!!!!
!

Make sure to keep the ball in a similar form throughout the entire exercise.

* Intensify and maintain the C curve of your spine

• Keep your abs tight

* Ensure that the buttocks are balanced by using abs

Be sure to keep your eyes on the belly button.

Make sure the heels are kept together and keep the toes separated.

* Remember your breath

Notes:

When you're dealing suffering from issues with their spines, like Scoliosis, it is not recommended to exercise this way. You could instead rolling up and down using knees bent as an exercise that is controlled.

Transition in Single leg stretch:

* Attach the ankle of the right side with your right hand

* Secure the right knee using the left hand.

* Wide elbows

Single leg stretch

5 ab series

Repetitions:

* 8-10 times per for each

Goals:

* Strengthening the abs

* Enhances coordination

* Strengthening legs

* Lengthening legs

* Increses stamina

Setting up:

* Straighten left leg 45 degree (from the ground) feet

in Pilates point

* Hold on to the lower right leg (or hold hands to

The mat is used to the mat to provide support)

* Slowly roll down, keeping the the shoulder blades and head from the

mat

*Look in the belly button

Make the exercise move:

* Breathe as you change legs

* Breathe in change legs, change and alter.

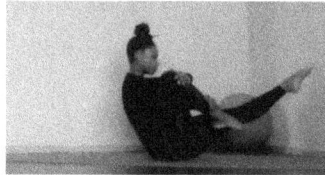

Corrections:

Make sure to keep the shoulders and head out of the mat.

* The straighter the lower leg, the further ahead.

* Hold on to the bent leg, bringing the leg to

The chest

* Push the abs into ensure they stay glued to your spine

Make sure your lower back is set to the mat! !

Be sure to keep an eye on the belly button.

* The straight leg's foot is placed in Pilates pointe (turned to the side)

Another foot is parallel to the other foot.

* Extending the straight line away

* The elbows remain broad shoulders.

• Keep your legs in close proximity to the middle of the body.

Keep reminding yourself of your breath

Notes:

The positions of arms is as follows;

* As you secure yourself to the lower leg of your right Your right hand should be at the ankle of the right leg, while the left hand rests on the knee of the leg on the right The elbows remain wide towards the side

If you switch legs, the left hand should be placed at the ankle of your left leg, and your right hand rests sitting on the knee of the left leg, your elbows are wide and towards the side.

Here is where you can train some arm leg coordination. For beginners, you'll be able to keep your knee in place using both hands. The more advanced the beginners become, they can learn the best hand position.

The direction in which your legs move really is contingent on if you're able to keep your lower back within the mat. This can be achieved through pulling your abs back and gluing them to the spine. Beginners should aim to extend your legs toward the ceiling and work in the proximal. As they advance, the further down the legs fall in working distal. The ideal is for the legs to be at to eye level.

Chapter 6: Change To Double Leg Stretch

* Both knees on the chest are held by the ankles

Double leg stretch

5 ab series

Repetitions:

* 8-10 times

Goals:

* Strengthening the abs

* Strengthening legs

* Lengthening legs

* Boosts endurance

The setup:

* Chest knees Hold the ankles

Start the exercise and move it:

* Breathe into straightening your legs and arms.

in the direction of travel at the same time.

* Rectangle the arms

* Breathe in knees towards the chest.

* Keep ankles in place

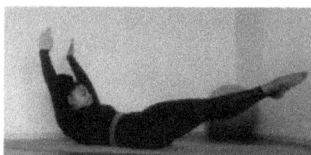

Corrections:

Be sure to keep an eye on the belly button.

• Keep your lower back firmly to the mat !!!! !

* Push the abs into ensure they stay firmly anchored to the spine

* The lower the leg, the more advanced

• Keep your shoulder and head off the mat.

* Straighten your arms close to your ear.

Reach your the legs and arms away as you'd like to be touched

adjacent walls

• Squeeze your buttocks as you extend the legs

* Remind yourself of the breath

Notes:

The direction in which your legs be really based on whether you're able to keep your lower back on the mat, by pulling your abs into by gluing your abs to the spine. For beginners, you'll want to extend your legs toward the ceiling and work in the proximal. As they advance, the further down the legs fall and work distal. Ideally, the legs should be placed at to eye level.

Transition in to Scissors:

* Both knees are in the chest.

Scissors

5 ab series

Repetitions:

* 8-10 times for each leg

Goals:

* Strengthening the abs

* Strengthening legs

* Lengthening legs

* Stretching your legs

* Boost Flexibility

* Stamina

Setting up:

* Simultaneously straighten left leg away 45 degrees

Straighten your right leg and point it towards the and straighten the right leg towards the nose

* Secure the left ankle

Start this exercise by moving it:

* Breath slowly and gently move right leg towards nose two times, pull it back.

* Breathe into Change legs, pull pull

* Adjust pull pull switch pull pull

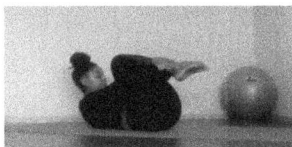

Corrections:

Continue to look in the belly button.

Make sure that the back is placed to the mat.

* Continue pulling your abs and keeping them in place to keep

spine

* Make sure the elbows are wide towards the side.

* The legs are bent out with feet in Pilates place.

69

Make sure that your legs are close to the centerline of your body.

Notes:

The way that your legs are able to move really is contingent on if you're able to keep your lower back firmly on the mat, by bringing your abs into the mat and gluing your abdominals to the spine. Beginners should aim to raise your legs toward the ceiling and work in the proximal. As they advance, and the more lower they go and work distal. The ideal is for the legs to be at to eye level.

If you find that your students are unable to grasp their ankles allow them to hold the calfs of their leg muscles, not their knees.

Transition to lower lift:

- Beginners

* The chest is swollen and knees are aching.

- Advanced beginner

* Legs straight up to the ceiling Pilates position.

Lower lift

5 ab series

Repetitions:

* 8-10 times

Goals:

* Strengthening the abs

* Strengthening legs

* Lengthening legs

* Strengthening the muscles of the butt.

* Stimulates endurance

The setup:

* Create a pillow for your hands.

Your hands should be placed in the behind your neck.

Straighten legs until the ceiling

* Feet turned in and legs out in Pilates place.

Make the exercise move:

* Breathe deeply and lower your legs toward
the mat 1,2,3.

* Breathe in and lift your legs and then lower
them back for 1 minute.

• Lower 3,3 higher as well.

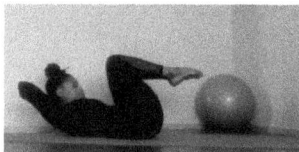

Corrections:

Make sure that the back is placed on the mat.

* Pull the abdominals into the spine to ensure
they are glued to the spine

Continue to look in the belly button.

* Make sure the elbows are wide and to the
side.

* Pull the muscles of but when you lower the leg.

to the mat

The lower the leg, the more advanced

Notes:

The direction in which your legs move depends upon whether you are able to keep your lower back firmly in the mat. This can be achieved by pulling your abs up and then gluing your spine to your abs. Beginners shouldn't have to lower your legs too significantly, working in distal. The further they progress, the more lower they go and work distal. The ideal is for the legs to be at to eye level.

The transition into Criss cross:

* Both legs to the ceiling

* Feet turned in and legs twisted out in Pilates place.

Criss cross

5 ab series

Repetitions:

* 8-10 times per for each

Goals:

* Strengthening abs, particularly the abs, and especially the obliques.

* Strengthening legs

* Lengthening legs

* Strengthening the muscles of the butt.

* Enhances endurance

The setup:

* Right knee to the chest with the parallel

Lower left leg, at 45° (from on the mat) Leg is turned out with the foot placed into Pilates position.

* Turn your body toward the knee bend.

* Wide elbows towards the side

Start the exercise and move it:

* Breathe in, and then change to the other side.

* Breathe into the change side.

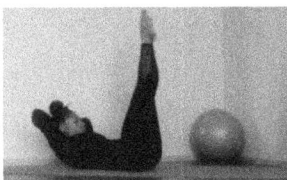

Corrections:

Make sure to keep the lower back firmly to the mat

Maintain the abs tight and secure to the spine.

* Continue lifting each shoulder blade out of the mat.

• Keep your legs in close proximity to the centerline of your body.

* Make sure the elbows are wide towards the side.

* Really stretch the straight leg

* Place both your hips on the mat.

* Twist your body away from to the waist

Notes:

The way that your legs are able to move really is contingent on whether you're able to keep the lower back on the mat, through pulling your abs back by gluing your abs to the spine. For beginners, you'll want to extend your legs towards the ceiling while working distal. As they advance, and the more lower they go in working distal. Ideally, the legs should be placed at in the eye.

Chapter 7: The Transition Into Spine Move Forward

* Both knees on the chest.

* Place the head back on the mat.

Advanced

* Both knees on the chest.

* Place the head back on the mat.

* Straighten your legs onto the mat. flex legs parallel

Arms to the ceiling

Spine stretch forward

Repetitions:

* 5 times

Goals:

• Increase spinal flexibility

* Flex the spine

Setting up:

Or, you can rock yourself until a seated posture, or hold your back to the

The thighs

Do a thorough roll-up similar to the exercise for rolling up to

The seated place

* The back is straight

* Legs as large as mat

* They are parallel to feet and can be flexed

"Arms reaching in forward the height of shoulders and shoulder height.

Width

Make the exercise move:

* Breathe in to make you higher.

* Breathe in and reach upwards and then over to the to the forward

* Retracting the spine in a straight forward breathe in

Corrections:

* Keep your abs and ribs tight

* Do not lift your shoulders.

* Lift the abs from your hips as you lift them up.

and above

Make sure to keep the arms ' shoulder height as well as wide at a minimum

reaching upwards and then to the side and

Make sure your feet are in a flex position and keep the legs active

It is an exercise of the spine, not the hamstrings.

Remember to keep reminding yourself of your breath

Note:

Imagine that you are climbing up to and over the top of a huge ball.

Transition into Open Leg rocker prepping:

* Whenever you are reaching to the top and above, secure your hands to your ankles

• Pull your feet toward you. As you roll upwards, knees are bent.

from the side. arms rest on the sides of the legs.

* Back straight

* Feet are located in Pilates place.

Open leg rocker prep

Repetitions:

* 10 second

* Or 10 counts

Goals:

* Strengthens the abs

Balance is improved

* Helps to focus

* Increases control

Setting up:

* Draw a tiny C curvature in the your lumbar spinal (lower back)

* Unlock the chest

Make the exercise move:

First, balance your feet on the mat. mat

* Straighten both legs (both simultaneously) or the other leg at the

time)

* Ensure that legs are shoulder width and straight

* and balance

Corrections:

* Maintain C curve in the lumbar spine

* Legs remain ahead of shoulders.

* Lift your chest.

* Look up at the horizon.

* Feet are at Pilates the correct position.

Straighten your arms.

* Shoulder to the side

Notes:

If your child isn't able move their legs in a straight line, let them in a bend. Concentrate more on the upper part of the body and the curve of C in the spine of the lumbar region, the focus and the equilibrium.

Transition in to Corkscrew:

* Lock the legs

* Letting go of the ankles and extend the arms in a parallel line

The legs

Corkscrew

Repetitions:

* 4 times each direction

Goals:

* Strengthening abs, particularly the abs, and especially the obliques.

* Strengthening legs

* Strengthening the muscles of the butt.

* Increases control

The setup:

* Create a curve through the spine.

* Check the belly button

* A spherical spine that runs down the mat

* Placed arms beside the one's body, the palms are towards the ground.

* Legs reach straight up to the ceiling

* With legs turned out and into Pilates place.

Start the exercise and move it:

* Breathe slowly in circles with your legs to the right

* Bring your legs back toward the center

* Breathe out in a circle, bringing the legs towards the left (opposite direction)

* Bring your legs back toward the center

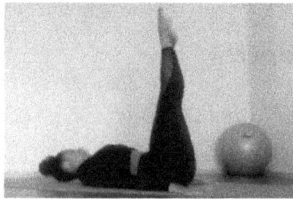

Corrections:

Make sure heels are kept together while you are circling your legs

* The butt may raise slightly, but the lower body will remain

The mat is still placed mat !!!! !

* Pull the buttocks to squeeze.

* Make sure that the hips remain still to the maximum extent possible.

* Kick the triceps towards the mat in order to stabilize the upper body.

* The ribs remain to the side

* Stretch the neck and head muscles.

* Bring the abs in ensure they stay glued to your spine

* Draw an image of a basketball in the ceiling (when

Advanced and more controlled think the skippy ball)

Make sure to keep your eyes on the ceiling

* Remember that breath

Notes:

The more advanced you are, the bigger the circle. Begin by drawing an orange across the ceiling, followed by the basketball, then the slippery ball. The better your control, the bigger circle.

Transition in to Saw:

* Slowly raise your legs and return to seated

* Legs are larger than mat

Saw

Repetitions:

* 5 times on each side

Goals:

* Extending the spine

* Increases flexibility of the spinal

* Extends the length of the spine.

Setting up:

* Sit in a position with legs that are wider than mat

* Back straight

* Both arms extend toward the side and palms downwards

* The legs that are parallel to the feet can be flexed

Start the exercise and move it:

* Breathe in and lift your hips to release the ribs. lower shoulders

* Twist the right from your waist

* Breathe in and reach upwards and back towards the pinky toe.

2,3

* The spine is articulated and backs up

Twist back around to the center breath in

* Repeat the same procedure on the reverse side

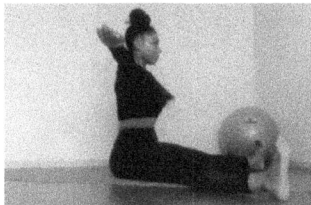

Corrections:

Make sure that both hips are on the mat. Keep them in a level position, especially during

You rotate the wheel to the left

Continue to lift up and up when you're reaching forward.

Imagine reaching out and over an enormous snowball

* Continue pulling your abdominals into

* While sitting straight, maintain the ribs and shoulders

down

* Remain flexible with your feet

• Keep your legs strong and Active.

Make sure the shoulder is lowered.

* Keep in mind your breath

Notes:

This isn't the form of a hamstring stretch. It is an exercise in spine rotation as well as a spine lengthening exercise. Reach over.

The transition the direction of Swan neck roll

* Close the legs

* Arms reach forward, shoulder height, length

* Pay attention to the stomach button curving in the spine.

* Begin by using the abs to roll onto the mat.

Swan neck roll

Repetitions:

* 3 times

2- Lift it up two times with no neck roll

3rd Time Neck Roll beginning right, and then reverse

Repeat the sequence 3 times.

Goals:

* The back is strengthened

* Increase the length of the spine.

* Stretching the abs

* Strengthening shoulders and arms

* Improves the flexibility of the neck

Setting up:

* Straighten your right leg and arm

* Bending left leg

* Force yourself to lie on your back (prone) upon the mat.

The mat's forehead lengthens the neck

* Hands are next to chest

* Elbows at the midsection of the

* Place feet on legs in Pilates the point

Make the exercise move:

Breathe into the forehead to lift it to lift the nose, lift chest, lift chin

* Push the hands

* Breathe into the spine and then to return back to the mat

Neck roll

* Make sure you look at the right

* Turn left and look down

• Look both ways.

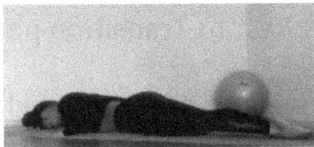

Corrections:

* Continue to engage the abs (pulling the abs away) from the

mat)

* Continue to squeeze the muscles of the but

* Always reach your legs to keep them away

* Make sure your elbows are in the mid-section of the

Maintain the length of your neck as you raise up the mat.

* Continue to squeeze your legs and heels

Notes:

Let your legs be to hip width apart, if your student is suffering from weak back or lower back issues.

Moving from Rest to Transition position:

* Put your weight on your ankles with the help of your hands

Chapter 8: The Resting Position

Repetition:

* Minimum 5 minutes (5 counts)

What ever length is necessary to keep the class moving of the class

to be considered

Goals:

* The counter stretch is a swan's neck the roll

* Stretching your lower back

* Short relaxing

Setting up:

* Open knees a bit

* Keep feet together

Start this exercise by moving it:

* Put a pushbutt onto the heels

* While curving the spine, you are by pulling abs back in

* Natural breath

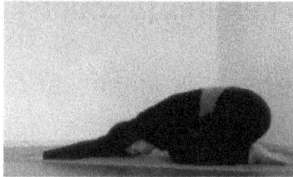

Correction:

* Continue to lift your abs toward the spine.

* Extend the abs from your thighs.

* Stay alert with this pose.

Make sure the arms are long and push the butt onto the

heels

* Make sure to keep the C curve within the spine in order to stretch the lower

to the back

Notes:

Maintain this posture so that you can maintain the flow of the class, and also to prevent your students from loosing energy.

It's still a very active position.

The transition into Shoulder bridge prepping:

* Roll all fours

* Place the toes on the mat

* Pull your hands away from you to engage the abs, turning the

the balls of your feet until you reach your feet to

Preparing the bridge for shoulder

Repetitions:

* Minimum 5 times

Goals:

• Strengthening the muscles in the butt.

* Facilitates articulation of spine

The setup:

* Bending knees

* Arms are reaching toward the forward

* Pay attention to your belly button, then roll back onto the mat.

* Bring your heels closer towards the but

* The feet and knees are held together by glue

* Arms reaching out in front of the the mat

The gaze is straight up toward the ceiling.

Make the exercise move:

* Breathe into the air, starting by releasing the butt/hips

* Articulate the spine upwards

* Breathe in and articulate the spinal column in the mat. lower back.

Lower back butt

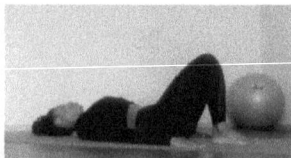

Corrections:

* Make sure to keep the abs and ribs in

Make sure to keep your chin from your chest.

* Put your hand onto the highest point

* They have as close to butt as you possibly can.

* Continue to reach your arms to the side of your body

* Abs and Butts kick off the beginning of the exercise.

The butt will be the only thing you'll find back on the mat, when you roll

to go back

Keep your hips at a single level. Imagine that you are balancing two tea bags

cups on either one side of your hip

* Keep in mind your breath

Notes:

Let your legs be to hip width apart, if your student is experiencing weak back or lower back issues.

Change to Side kicks in the front and back

Straighten the left leg and right arm

* Push yourself up to the right side by using the left bend

Leg

Kicks in the side, front and back

Side kick series

Repetitions:

* 5-10 times

Goals:

* Strengthening the legs as well as butt muscles.

* Lengthening legs

* Strengthening the abs

Focus and control

The setup:

* Lay on your back aligning yourself towards the back of your

mat

Straight to the back

* The right hand is supporting the left hand of the head in the front of

Your chest should be into the mat in order to help stabilize your posture. Place your chest in the mat to stabilize it.

* Place your legs a bit ahead of you on the mat

* Flexing the left leg and foot onto the mat

* Lifting left leg with the hips to the side, foot is Pi

lates point

Start the exercise and move it:

* Breathe into kick kick forward

* Breathe in kick, kick in and then return

* As well as Kick kick (front) as well as kick kick (back)

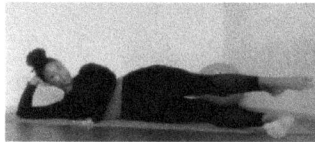

Corrections:

* Engage the abs and then push them into the hands onto the mat until

stabilize the body position

Start the kicks with the Powerhouse

Maintain upper and hips as steady as you can.

Keep your legs at a in the hips when kicking forward and back.

Continue to push on the heels (of the leg on the mat) towards the mat.

mat. Keep lengthening the heel.

* Make sure to keep the leg of the leg on top turned with feet directed

Maintain a long neck and straight with the

spine

Keep extending both legs. Both legs are working.

* Continue lifting your body's waist off the mat.

* Remember that breath

Notes:

2 tiny kicks rear and front.

The greater the distance that a leg can go is contingent on how stable and steady the hips are as well as the flexibility of the person doing the exercise. The exercise does not concern how high the legs go it's about how steady the hips and upper body are while removing both legs out of the powerhouse. This workout is about being in control.

Then, transition to Side Kicks Up & Down:

* Heels join together

Make sure that the top leg is in place and keep the lower leg is parallel

and was flexed to push it into and out of

Side kicks up and down

Side kick series

Repetitions:

* 5-10 times

Goals:

* Strengthening legs and butt muscles.

* Increasing the length of legs

* Strengthening the abs

* Stretching your legs

It helps focus and maintain control.

Setting up:

* Heels in a row

• Keep the top leg in place and keep the lower leg in line

and then flexed in and out of

Start the exercise and move it:

* Breathe through the lift leg until it reaches ceiling.

* Breathe deeply and pull your to bring your

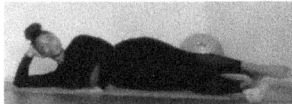

leg down

Corrections:

* Begin the leg motion using the Powerhouse

* Make sure that the upper part of your body is completely still.

* Make sure the hips remain still and centered.

* Keep the upper leg straight, turned and straight with the keep the foot inside.

Pilates point

* Continue to push the heel of your bottom leg into the mat.

Make sure the neck is longer and your head straight.

* Remember to breathe.

Notes:

The more high the leg rises will depend on how level and still your hips are as well as the flexibility of the person doing the exercise. The exercise does not concern how high you can lift your leg, it's about how well it is possible to resist your leg as it goes down, and how level the hips and upper back are.

This workout is about being in control. You can also stretch your foot while putting the leg downwards.

Then transition to Side kick circles

* Heels are joined

• Keep the top leg in place and keep the lower leg in line

and was flexed to push it into and out of

Side kicks circles

Side kick series

Repetition:

* 5-10 times each direction

Goals:

* Strengthening legs and butt muscles.

* Lengthening legs

* Strengthening the abs

* Extend the legs

It helps focus and maintain control.

Setting up:

* Heels are joined

Make sure that the top leg is left out, and the bottom leg is parallel

and was flexed to push it into and out of

Make the exercise move:

* Breathe into circle in forward, upwards, back

Breathe in and bring your bring your heels back

*, circle, and circle, etc.

* Invert the circles

Correction:

* Make sure to keep the heels while circling

Maintain the upper lower body as well as the hips and legs still.

Start the motion by removing the Powerhouse

* Make sure to keep the abs and ribs kept in

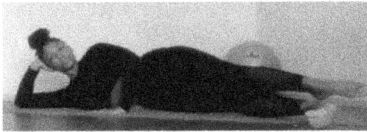

* Make sure that the leg which is in a circle turned and feet

Pointed

* Push the heel of the lower leg into the mat.

* Picture drawing your own grapefruit onto the wall

* Keep in mind that breath

Notes:

The more advanced, the larger the circle. Begin by creating a picture of a grapefruit on the wall. Next, imagine drawing an basketball, and finally the skippy ball. The better your control, the bigger the circle.

Then, transition into Side kicks the thigh's internal lift upwards and downwards:

* Heels joined

Make sure that the top leg is in place and keep the lower leg in line

and was flexed to push it into and out of

Side kicks lift the inner thigh both up and down

Side kick series

Repetitions:

* 5-10 times

Goals:

* Strengthening legs and butt muscles.

* Lengthening legs

* Strengthening the abs

* Extend the legs

It helps focus and maintain control.

Setting up:

* Move left leg until the ceiling

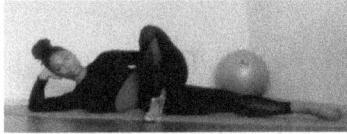

* Place the left foot between the hips.

• Through the open in the leg, secure the ankle

* Letting the right leg to long the mat, pointing your foot

As well as parallel

Start the exercise and move it:

* Breathe deeply and lift the right leg

* Breathe and resist the one leg

Corrections:

Start leg movements with the Powerhouse

* Hold your upper body and thighs still.

* The neck lengthening is straight

Continue to lengthen the bottom leg, and continue to reach

farther away, as you lower your leg

* Make sure left foot is planted to the mat

* Keep in mind your breath

Notes:

If the student isn't able to bend his left leg in the manner shown in the photo above, you can place the knee bent on the mat, supported by an object like a pillow or another prop.

Change to side kicks the inner thighs in circles

* Make sure your leg is to be ready for a circle

Side kicks and inner thighs circle

Chapter 9: Side Kick Series

Repetitions:

* 5 times each direction

Goals:

* Strengthening legs and butt muscles.

* Increasing the length of legs

* Strengthening the abs

* Stretching your legs

It helps focus and maintain control.

Setting up:

* Through the opening in the leg, hold onto the ankle

* Reaching for the right leg up (Just completed up and down)

Make sure you keep your leg in place)

Start the exercise and move it:

* Breathe out in circle, the front, back, lower

* Breathe deeply and your leg will be back up

*, circle, * and circle.

* Invert the circles

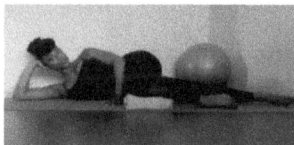

Corrections:

* Start the leg movements by utilizing the Powerhouse

Maintain the upper lower body as well as the hips and legs still.

* Longening the neck to ensure that the it is straight.

Continue to lengthen the bottom leg, and continue to reach

more while you are the aircraft circles

* Keep your left foot fixed to the mat.

* Remember your breath

Notes:

With this exercise, you'll be able to build the circle as wide as you can while keeping the stability of your hips and the upper part of your body.

Change to Beats to the belly.

Place both legs on the top of one another

The heels together continue to lift each leg off the mat

Beats in the stomach

Exercise to transition into right side kick sequence left

Repetitions:

* 20 beats

Goals:

* Intensifying the inner thighs

* Transferring to the series of side kicks to the left side to the left side.

The left side

The setup:

* Switch on the belly

* Continue to lift your legs away from the mat.

* Turn legs to the side and feet placed remain in Pilates heel point.

Together

* Create a pillow from your hands, and then allow your forehead to rest

in your hands

* Pulling your abs off the mat and towards the spine.

Start the exercise and move it:

* Lift and close the legs

"Touching heels each at certain times

*, and a beat beat (tempo is quite fast)

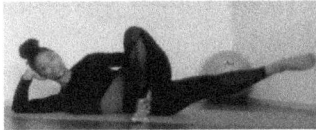

Corrections:

* Lift your abs away from the mat toward the

spine

* Continue lifting your legs off the mat.

* Press the muscles of your butt.

Make sure the neck is length

Continue to lengthen your legs.

• Keep your body as still as is possible just the
legs.

Moving

* Natural breath

Repetition all of the side kicks sitting on your
left side

• Turn to the left and prepare for side kicks both front and back

The transition into Teaser One leg

* Place each leg on top of one another.

• Then, you can place the leg with the highest bend in front of you.

* Push yourself up to an upright position, or a standing position.

lying on the floor

* The right leg is bent while the left leg remains straight. Knees are

Together

Teaser one leg

Repetitions:

* 5 times per leg

Goals:

* Strengthening abs

* Strengthening legs

Focus and control

* Increases the spinal flexibility

Setting up:

* Sit down.

* The right leg is bent feet straight on the floor, parallel

* Left leg straight and turned inwards, with feet are in Pilates position.

* Knees are held together by glue.

* Push bend leg further away from the butt, while keeping the knees

Together

* Arms reaching forward on the diagonal direction, parallel to

Straight leg

C-curve into the spine and an unlocked chest

* Look out to the horizon.

Start the exercise and move it:

* Breathe in and look towards the belly button.

Breathe deeply as you slide down

* Move arms in front of the ears. Place ribs inside

* Breathe in and then look up in belly roll

• Reach your arms out diagonally to the side, and then open your chest.

look upwards

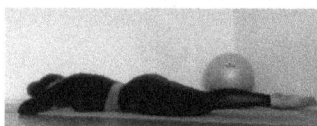

Corrections:

* Keep your knees to one another for the duration of the workout.

* If you are reaching your arms behind next to ears, hold the ribs inside

Maintain the abs kept in place and glued to your spine.

* While rolling, keep checking your the belly button

Keeping the C curve within the spine

* While rolling, keep your eyes on the belly button.

Keeping the C curve within the spine

* When you reach the highest level, look upwards and then start the

chest

* Continue to keep aiming to the straight leg

* Keep in mind your breath

Notes:

You should really take the time to examine the two distinct sets ups and transitions to the Teaser one segment. It is possible to take a time before beginning Teaser I. Start by placing both knees on the chest, then lower the head back. The ideal is to keep going straight into this Teaser I after the Teaser one leg. It's a tough workout, so you must be focused on how you perform this practice. Make sure you are using your best phrases.

Transition in to Teaser I:

Straight legs, reaching out 45 degrees away from the

mats inside Pilates point

Teaser I

Repetitions:

* 5 times

Goals:

* Strengthening abs

* Strengthening your legs

Focus and control

* Improves flexibility in the spine.

Setting up:

* Sit in a comfortable posture.

* Both legs are 45 degrees away from the mat

* Legs are straight and feet are placed in Pilates position.

* Reaching your arms diagonally and parallel to the legs

Create a C-curve around the spine.

* Looks toward the horizon with an unlocked chest

Make the exercise move:

* Breathe in and look towards the belly button.

Breathe in as you turn in the opposite direction.

* Move arms in front of the ears. Place ribs inside

Breathe in and then look up in belly roll

* Move arms and arms diagonally in the direction of forward. Open your chest

look at the sky

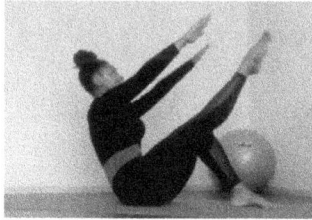

Corrections:

Make sure the heels are glued all the time

* As you reach your arms back, hold the spine in

Maintain the abs held in a tight position and secure to the spine.

* When you're rolling down, continue eyeing your the belly button

Keeping the C curve within the spine

* While rolling, keep eyeing the belly button.

Keeping the C curve within the spine

* Once you have reached the top spot, you should look to the left and take the time to open the

Chest

Keep aiming for the legs to stay away

* Pull the muscle of the butt.

* Keep in mind that breath

Notes:

This exercise can be left out if the students do not possess the strength they need yet. Start using the Teaser just one leg until they've developed the stamina and strength.

In the transition to Swimming preparation:

* When you've rolled down on the Teaser I, you'll go straight into

The change

* Right leg and right arm standing straight onto the mat

* Bending left leg, foot is parallel to with the mat

* Left hand positioned next to your body, pull your body to an upright position.

Position

Chapter 10: Preparation For Swimming

Repetitions:

* Three times on each side

Goals:

* Lengthens spine

* Strengthening the back muscles

Setting up:

* Lie prone

* Straight arms in front of the ears

* Stretch the entire body the opposite direction.

* Turning legs together with feet to Pilates position.

* Forehead on mat with long neck

Make the exercise move:

* Breathe deeply and lift the right leg and left arm simultaneously.

* Breath in lengthening legs and arm back into the mat

simultaneously

* Repeat with the other arm and leg

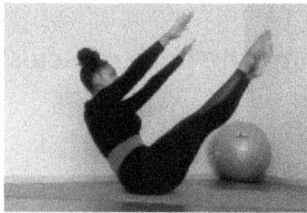

Corrections:

* Continue lifting your abs away from the mat.

Continue to squeeze the muscles of the butt

Make sure that the legs are near to the middleline when lifting the

Leg to and from

* Make sure that the hip bones remain on the mat.

* Neck is long

* Make sure that your legs are turned out, and the feet firmly in Pilates position.

* Make sure the body is still in a straight line, with no side-to-side movement.

* Keep lengthening in opposite direction

Transition in to Swimming:

* Lower your legs and arms into the mat.

* Forehead on the mat

Swimming

Repetitions:

* 10-12 times

Goals:

* Lengthens spine

* Strengthening the back muscles

* Improves the control of the body

The setup:

* Lie prone

* Arms straight to the ears

* Stretch the entire body the opposite direction.

* Turning legs together with feet to Pilates position.

* Forehead on mat with long neck

Make the exercise move:

* Pull both arms and legs out of from the mat.

* We also swim in the pool, swim and more swim. (Alternating

the opposite leg, and arm moving up and up and)

* Natural breath

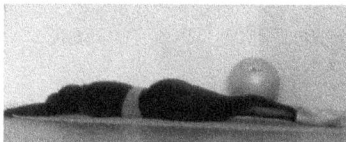

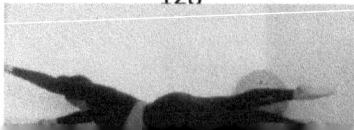

Corrections:

* Continue lifting your abs off the mat.

* Continue to squeeze butt muscles.

• Keep your legs in line with the centreline as you lift the leg

and to the down

* Make sure that the hip bones remain on the mat.

* Neck length stays

* Make sure your legs are turned and feet firmly in Pilates place.

* Make sure your body isn't turning from side to side

* Keep lengthening in opposite direction

Transition to leg Pull front support

* Lower your legs as well as arms into the mat.

* Forehead on the mat

Front support for leg pull (plank)

Repetitions:

* 10 sec- 1minute

Goals:

* Strengthening the abs

* Arms strengthening

* Strengthening the shoulders

The setup:

* Now, dig toes into the feet of your mat (or when in Pilates position)

Place hands on chest

* Elbows are glued to the waist

* Forehead is in matlong neck

Start the exercise and move it:

* Lift yourself up to a your plank posture (by pushing the

hands with 1 movement)

* Long neck

* Hold

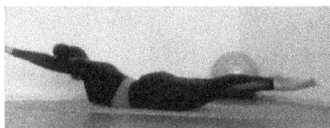

Corrections:

* Lift to your plank with one hand similar to a stiff board.

* Tighten the muscles around your butt slightly by tucking your hips inwards

* Continue pushing lower back towards the ceiling

* Pull abs to ensure they stay glued to spine

* Keep neck length

Continue to lengthen throughout the entire spinal

* The feet and legs are positioned parallel (or Pilates stance)

* You could have the feet and legs together, or have a hip length

Apart from that

Notes:

If your child isn't sufficient to raise them upwards to plank in a single move, they should put their knees in the ground and climb up to plank, keeping their knees to the mat.

Chapter 11: Change To Mermaid Stretch

* Place the right knee onto the mat, knee towards the other direction.

from the mat

* Bend your left knee, then sit on the buttocks of your right side.

* Both knees bent to the left side of the body.

Mermaid stretch

Repetitions:

* 3-4 times on each for each

Goals:

* Extends the sides of the body.

* Stretches the hip

Setting up:

Sit primarily on right buttocks

The legs are bent in front of one another on the left of

The body

* Secure ankles using left hand

* Hold right hand straight up to ceiling and glued over your ear

* Shoulders to the side

Start the exercise and move it:

* Breathe out in length and extend the hips and ribs

* Breathe in and reach upwards and down towards the left of your the body.

* Breathe in, then come all the way back straight, with both arms in the

the other side

* Now, reach left hand to ceiling and bind to the ear

* Breathe and lift up and then over to the right side of the

Body, placing the left arm on mat

* Breathe in and come in straight arms.

the other side

The mermaid should be able to transition in the buttocks on the left:

Place your hands behind your back

* Tighten the legs on the right of the body.

Repeat the exercises on the other side.

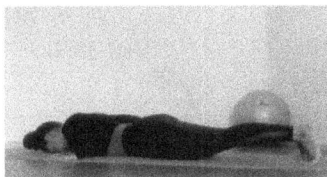

Corrections:

* Continue lifting your ribs away from the hips, focusing on the

the person who is reaching up to and the top

Imagine a person going across and up a large snowball

Maintain your shoulders in a straight line as you raise your arm.

ceiling

* The goal is to ensure that both cheeks of the butt off the mat.

Continue to push back toward the opposite buttocks.

* Keep in mind that breath

Transition in to Seal:

• Put your hands in front of you.

* Bring the legs up to the side of the mat.

Seal

Repetitions:

* 8 times

Goals:

* Strengthens the abs

* Cooldown

• Massage the spinal column

* Clapping your feet could open up energy blockages within the body, and also stimulates the circulation of blood

The setup:

* Sit down with your feet joined with your knees extending toward the sides

* Keep your hands on the foot's outside and then move through the

The gap between the legs

Create a C-curve of your spine while lifting both feet off the ground.

The mat

* Pay attention to the stomach

Ab muscles are pulled into and glued to the spine

Make the exercise move:

* Clap your feet 2,3 (clap feet three times)

* Breathe deeply, the back of your head and then make a clap of 2,3.

* Breathe deeply to move up and then balance

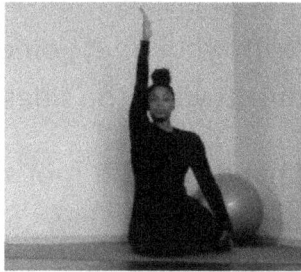

Corrections:

* Always keep an eye on the stomach

* Continue to pull abs into the abdominals, thereby launching the rolling back

From the abs

Maintain your C curve within the spine

* Roll on your shoulder blades. Keep the head in place and

Neck out of mat!! !

* Hold the entire foot

* Make sure the shoulders are down

Notes:

If you are a person with back issues like scolioses, it is not recommended to perform this workout. You can instead perform a roll-up and down with the knees bent in a controlled workout called crunching.

Change into the Push-up series:

When you have completed the last Seal Roll back

* Allow the feet to move through one motion and then bring them to a standing position.

the position

If you are able, but if you cannot make use of hands

in order to rise to the level of standing

* Reverse the ball and feet so that they face towards the higher end of the

Mat

* Make an Pilates position

Chapter 12: Series Of Push-Ups

Repetitions:

* 3 times

Goals:

* Strengthen the abs

* Strengthen your shoulders and arms.

The setup:

* Make the Pilates position

* Moving the arms toward the ceiling

* Shoulder back with abs, ribs and shoulder were pulled into

Make the exercise move:

* Roll to articulate the spine

* Lay your hands lying flat on the floor, ideal legs remain straight

(bend legs, if necessary)

* Walk 3 steps while using the hands in the plank in a seated

• Push one push up, 3. (breathe into when

Pushing down, exhale while pushing upwards

* Raise the butt until it reaches the ceiling (downwards towards the dog)

* Walk the hands in three steps back.

* Bringing the spine into a standing position,

Pilates Stance

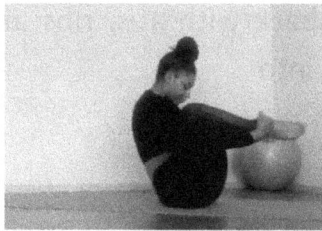

Corrections:

* Maintain your feet in Pilates position, and keep the your heels in place

* Pull the abs to keep them in

* When you roll down the you can articulate your spine

In the plank position, continue pressing the back of your upper body towards

The ceiling

* Pull the muscles of your butt to plank. Push to the side.

the position

* Make sure the elbows are in the waist during push ups.

* Long neck plank in long neck in push-up position, and a downwards

Facing dog

* Keep in mind your breath

Notes:

If you feel that your students aren't capable of doing the push ups, they should put on their knees while doing the push-up or allow them to lower their knees while holding the position.

End in a solid Pilates posture.

All of these are Classical Pilates mat beginners exercises. Take the time to study the images from this book, as well as those of YouTube. YouTube Channel Classical Pilates. I hope you have enjoyed the Classical Pilates journey so far.

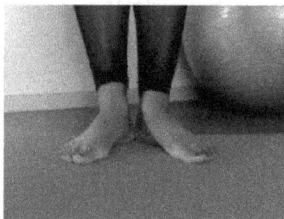

8. Terminology List

Pilates position (feet bent, two fists in between the toes)

The ballet first position (Legs are extended to the maximum extent they are able without bending the legs. Keep them straight and straight back. Knees are pointed towards the same direction as toes)

Feet running parallel

Aim for a straight line with your feet parallel to hip width (2 fingers between heel and the

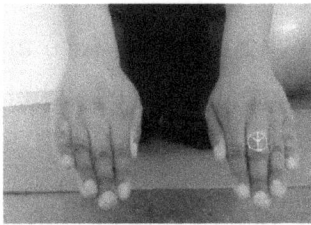

toes)

Pilates place (heels together)

Flexible feet

Foots with pointed toes

All fours (Arms straight underneath the shoulder and knees straight beneath the hips)

Put your toes into the mat

The chest is swollen and knees are aching.

Table top knees (knees 90o)

A C curve of spine

Straight back/flat rear

Seal exercises (arms are placed in the space between knees and hold to feet)

Side kicks: In the thigh lift (use an object or a cushion beneath the knee when your child can't get into the right posture)

Pilates hand place (fingers to each other, during the majority of exercises)

Prone (lying with face down)

Supine (lying on the floor with your face facing up)

Chapter 13: Scientifically Acceptable Reasons As Well As Other Reasons Why

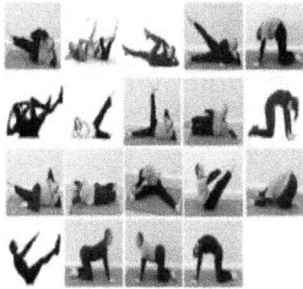

Pilates Is Amzing

The scientifically proven the reasons Pilates can be a complete path towards inner harmony and overall health, are as follows:

1. Pilates helps to improve your brain and helps you become more savvy.

In our 20s, most of us start losing about 1% of the amount of our hippocampus. It is an area of our brain that is responsible for memory and cognitive capacity. The cerebrum is in a actual sense contracted.

In the past, researchers thought that we were born to the planet with specific numbers of synapses, however recently they discovered that the cerebrums of our brain could create new cells, which could then dial back or shrinking the brain's switching. What are the implications for your life? This could mean greater memory, less risk of developing Alzheimer's disease, improved understanding and critical thinking and a greater IQ and sky's the limit. Recent studies show that increased activity enhances neurogenesis. These changes are usually visible in the hippocampus. This is which is the location responsible for memory and the process of learning.

A different group of professionals at University of Illinois at Urbana-Champaign. University of Illinois at Urbana-Champaign says that individuals are prone to having a predominant cerebrum activity after a meticulous training routine like Pilates or Yoga when contrasted with intense exercise.

2. Pilates prepares your cerebrum. The process of learning new exercises can be a

proven cerebrum preparation method. In one study, it was discovered that completing new tasks increases the size of the cerebrum's white matter (the filaments which allow neurons to transmit.) If the neurons are designed but they aren't interfacing, eventually they will die without any benefit to mental well-being, therefore this white matter is crucial.

Moving your body is essential to brain health. Yet, many of us do not have extra few hours each week to decide the best way to move around or embark to a new leisure pursuit.

The activity plan is a great way to accomplish a variety of tasks and help our body as well as our mental health at the same time. When you are ready to begin your workout (like doing a run and sitting at the television, or doing a few repetitions in the center of the exercise without focusing in on your form or going through the same Yoga set-up each week) your gains are cut of exercise by fifty-fifty. but not at all, noting that you double the risk of having an issue with your physical health.

Based on a study, making a change or making a change to the Pilates routine is not enough to provide what we're looking to achieve by testing our mind and body simultaneously.

3. A more profound muscle activation implies more capacity for the sensor system.

When we move, there are a handful of specific places in our minds. The cerebrum after that, initiates an impulse through the spinal line and into muscles filaments. The process is more complicated than this and demands an additional packing.

When you discover how to sincerely connect with a specific muscles (like the profound actuation of the center in Pilates) you trigger an entrainment chain that could had been asleep for some time. Did you know that the center of your body is comprised of 29 muscles along with an oblique six-pack?

Finding out ways to use the 29 muscles can be a cleanse to your senses.

A strong sensory system means more communication between your mind and the different parts of your body, as well as you begin to experience the effects of stress and mind-set enhancing chemical.

4. Relax your mind and feel good through Pilates.

There is a good chance that you have read a great deal about the benefits of taking care reflection to the body and your brain. These benefits can be described as:

It reduces misery and anxiety.

-helps treat a sleeping disorder,

The brain is honed

It uncovers the most innovative thinking,

-diminishes pressure

assists with the ongoing torture of management,

It reduces the negative feeling

Helps fight addictions and reinforce positive tendencies

It is a great way to reduce your pulse and boost the cardio-vascular well-being.

If a majority people think on this topic, we think of the image of a Buddhist priest or New Age individual reciting in the solitude. But, perhaps we're out of our element when we think of the one method by which we can the concept of care could be incorporated into our daily routine of living.

Pilates helps you focus your attention on aspect of your body. No matter if you need it, it is essential to clear one's head of any distractions in case you're practicing Pilates harmony exercises on the Reformer, or for the second time if it is just the internal spring inside your center, which your instructor is discussing.

Pilates lets you enjoy each of the advantages of contemplation, without having to stand on the sidelines and feeling like that you're wasting the time you have.

Benefits from care can be obtained as long as you're comfortable with your actions. Many people enjoy the peace of meditation, while others benefit from the careful process of purging the brain when they practice by using their body.

5. Pilates diminishes pressure strain in our body.

It is likely that you have heard of the well-known "instinctive" reaction to upsetting situations. If you are confronted the adversity of a situation (genuine similar to being into a car accident or a novel, similar to anxiety about public speaking) your body produces an influx of stress chemicals that prime the body to fight or flee.

If we're in an uncomfortable situation, the body will perform at the highest level However, in most circumstances, we aren't able to escape when stuck in an awkward situation and also shouldn't trigger our primary. Work that is active should take advantage of the production of stress-related chemicals but we are able to stay inside the situation and handle the situation.

The result? Stress chemicals may trigger muscle cramps, hypertension and pain.

Pilates eases tension in muscles via gentle stretching and a progressive mold. An intense exercise on the Jump Board can help you process the pressure-related chemicals that are produced in the muscles. Additionally, the fascial release methods that a lot of Pilates instructors employ during their class today can aid in relaxing muscles that aren't open to extending and dissociating. When you are worried about your body, you also ignore the body.

An untroubled body free of stress and weak is the perfect sanctuary basically to settling an even brain that is capable of taking on all the complexities of modern daily life.

6. Pilates and Yoga help you reduce your stress.

What can you do to alleviate stress on your body and prevent tension from entering the brain? If you do not take care of the cause for your pressure (the method by which you perceive situations and respond to these) there isn't the possibility of having a long-lasting ease of pressure.

Yoga and Pilates shows demonstrate a relentlessness and ease, they teach the body to recognize resistance within the body and utilize this to manage your body. A different study revealed the benefits of reducing pressure of a traditional and surprising only-once Yoga gathering. According to the authors that the test for the posture is what could be described as the stressor. This is what happens in the course of a Pilates class which joins half-way and moves through Pilates exercises or focuses on the stream of progress. When the actual needs are addressed with regular breathing, the system of sensory responds, keeping pace with the ebb and flow while maintaining the feeling of a calm. This lets us face our daily stress with clarity and to respond without becoming overwhelmed.

7. Pilates helps you be more happy.

In the event that you enjoy Pilates and it makes your life more enjoyable.

In the moment that the body's nervous system is heightened as it is during a favorite exercise, the hormones called endorphins enter the body which make us be more comfortable. When you engage in fitness and stay focused in it, instead of the mind wandering in other directions, you'll be happy and calm towards the finish. Real wellness is the most important requirement for happiness.

8. Pilates helps you become more creative.

The ability to think creatively and openly lets us face life in a whole new way and come up with innovative strategies for dealing with life's challenges.

Training and reflection have been proven the ability to develop innovation. If you combine the two during an Pilates exercise, you'll more favorable outcomes to your mental health and body.

9. Pilates helps you control your emotions.

The way we feel and the quality of our breathing is closely linked. The results of a recent study revealed that a variety of states of excitement have a direct connection to breathing patterns. Take note of how your breathing alters as you encounter something shocking instead of a wonderful thing. It's not a significant improvement in this discovery just a matter of being aware.

However, the most interesting part of the review was that the distinctive breath examples trigger specific feelings. Inhale to a state of ease or annoyance.

The most important thing is to discover how to breathe successfully.

Breath is among the essential six Pilates guidelines. Learning to manage your breathing is one of the biggest benefits of Pilates as a lot of us are referred to as "sluggish breathers". Techniques you will learn during the Pilates class could also be applied in a variety of situations to help you relax or get through a difficult situation.

10. Careful Movement helps discharge enthusiastic pressure.

A psyche or body skill can reveal the character of yours simply by looking at the way you stand and your growth. In the long run, you store your emotions and tensions inside our body. Our jaws are clenched when you need to shout. We slump when we are feeling mediocre or modest, then fix our hips in order to block out the feelings of sadness and dread.

Pilates exercise helps you relax the muscles and control the core muscles which can most of the time become firmly linked to the weight of your mind. When you release muscles that are holding the tension of your life, you also release the mental burden you've carried about for no matter what amount of time.

11. Pilates allows you to behave naturally. In the modern world, it puts us under a number of demands as we are constantly trying to conform to certain rules. It is always necessary push ourselves to fulfill a limit, become a better child or watch the latest demonstrations according to the latest methods. Pilates helps us see the body as worthy and to be content with that body. It is all about exercising within your range of exercise and fostering your endurance and apprehension consistently. It is incredibly fascinating. When you are confident about what we're doing, you will find motivation and strength to take it towards a greater level. However, we aren't encouraged by the

comparison of ourselves to other people, but rather by establishing our own rules and expectations that are crucial for us.

Once we learn to view our bodies in the way we do, we determine how we can do similarly with the various different things we do. The way we live our lives is determined by our desires and needs instead of being aware about the Joneses.

Pilates is all about a great posture and a proper body alignment. Of course, a great posture is crucial for a healthy body, however, you'll also gain an advantage that is certain and helps you to become more confident and firm.

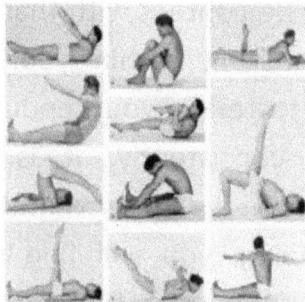

Chapter 14: Pilates Principles You Should Know

What is it that is

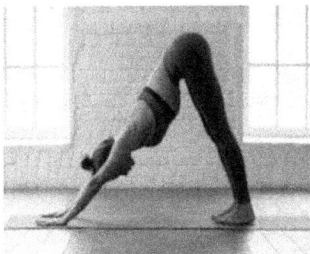

Get your rec-focus mat and prepare for a series of progress that can adapt and also to support your center.

The exercise is usually conducted with a particular solicitation each one following the other. They are referred to by names for instance "The 100," Criss-Cross," the "Elephant," and"The "Swan." They may appear simple however they require an immense amount of precision and the ability to control. While doing lots of crunches, there's an emphasis on the strategy. It is possible to do Pilates using the mat with an action as a group or at home with Pilates guidelines that are which are explained in this fantastic tutorial. You may go to a recreation centre or studio which has incredible equipment, a class or even a teacher who will supervise your progress.

The typical Pilates class lasts about 45 to 60 minutes however, you are able to do smaller movements faster than what you'd expect.

You'll be more stable and tense muscles and also improve the flexibility. It is possible to achieve better posture and enjoy the sensation of thriving that is unbeatable.

You should plan to do this exercise every two to three days in addition to your cardio as Pilates doesn't have the most amazing results.

Power Level: Medium

The activity is mentioned, but it's not an activity that consistently consumes real calories. All things revolve around the center, and then it's not winding. You'll be able to feel the tension in your muscles with any move.

Areas It Targets

In the end, you want to experience strength increases on the arms, as well as legs. Improvements and positions that are used to establish focus depend on cutting-off points for control and also apply loads.

Type

Versatility: Yes. Exercises within an Pilates workout will improve the flexibility of your joints as well as flexibility of joints.

Lively: No. It's not a cardio workout. out.

Strength: Yes. It will increase your muscle strength and help you stay grounded. It will be using your own body weight, not the weight of a load.

Sport: No.

Low-Impact: Yes. The muscles you pull at will attract with a powerful, yet delicate way.

Benefits and benefits from Pilates

There are therapeutic and shield benefit of Pilates due to the fact that it relaxes and loosens the muscles that are overworked; it also strengthens it with breath control and control. This can also provide you with more power and aids in executing your plans by assisting you in your plan. It also alters your posture and makes you be more upright and strong.

As with yoga, perhaps its greatest advantage is the growth and development that may result out from feeling much better as research shows. The bracing of your midriff and may help reduce discomfort due to the fact that it is more aside from tight muscles, it can ease lower back pain can result due to misalignment or lack of strength.

Pilates also provides additional body massage, it also helps to improve. When we accept that we are rehearsing, and then kicking the frame off and assisting our muscles you'll feel better. In addition, this could keep your aching lower back.

Yet, there are studies that show there are two requirements. The most important thing is to ensure that you are supervised by a certified instructor. If it's an individual or as part of an event with friends you should make sure it's at your level, and you increase the challenge consistently. It's not a matter of ricocheting in the direction of your teacher. They must recognize the problem.

In addition, it is recommended to complement the exercise with different training that is not Pilates. This isn't a totally free exercise. Because you're exercising your muscles it will bring your heart rate increased, but it's not the same as a cardiovascular workout. If you're facing an obstacle, but this is essential to the exercise routine to be even.

Chapter 15: Great Pilates Exercises That'll Work Your Core From Any Angle With No Equipment

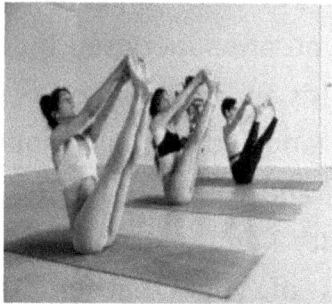

Pilates Exercises That Improve Your Core From Every Angle not Including Any Equipment

Being able to have a strong center is essential to stay well-balanced from the top up to your feet. So when you're looking to strengthen your core by incorporating the Pilates routine (or more than two!) in your weekly workout routine is a remarkable strategy. Perhaps the most significant benefit of Pilates is the ability to build stability and endurance at the waist area.

Additionally, you could gain these benefits without equipment aside from the exercise mat. Here are fifteen Pilates exercises that I believe will help you build an enduring foundation to strengthen your core (for for instance, abdominals as well as back).Regardless however, if you're unable to attend the class, you could at any time use these moves to build your own at-home Pilates practice that tests your core from every angle.

This exercise is suitable to all fitness levels. Please follow my suggestions below and I wish you the best of luck! you!

Timing: 25-30 minutes

Gear: mat

Useful for: center, abs

Instructions: Perform the suggested number of sets aswell in reps for every exercise and then move on towards the next activity.

Spanning

The best method for begin is to lie on your back with your legs bent and with feet flat on the floor, and arms at sides. Turn tailbone over and then lift effortlessly off flooring, and then lift every vertebra until the middle structure straightens across shoulders and knees. Take a break at the top to slam glutes. Alternate movements to start. It's one repetition. Perform two sets comprising 10 reps.

Stomach Curl

Instructions for step-by-step Begin lying back with legs turned with feet flat on the ground, arms in front of shoulders, arms wide. Intensify abs, lower jawline a bit, then turn neck, head and shoulders from the mat in specific arrangement. Then, gradually reverse the movements until you return to the starting point. It's one repetition. Do two sets with 10 repetitions.

Taps on the toes

Instructions: Lay on the back, with arms to side, legs bent at 90 degrees with feet raised to the sky so that your they are parallel to the flooring. Pivot on the hip joint, bringing lower left foot to the floor, but not letting your lower back slip away from mat. Return the leg to its starting place by connecting your abs to the lower. It's a single repetition. Perform two sets of 10 reps on each side.

Bike

A great way to do this is begin lying back with the hands on top of your shoulders and arms wide and legs bent at 90 degrees and feet elevated in the air to ensure that the shins align with the floor. While doing this, you can pivot your middle to the right-hand side and expand while forgetting about the leg directly at the 45-degree angle. Maintain your hips in a straight line when you move your body. Return to your starting point and switch sides. It's one rep. Do two sets of 20 repetitions.

The best method for start lying on your the right side, bending according to hips left leg bent so that your heel aligns with butt. Laying on the floor. Left leg stretched straight out in the air, aligned with the flooring. Lift left leg about two inches, then revisit. This is one repetition. Perform two sets with 20 reps each side.

Mollusk

Most effective way to start lying on the side with legs bent to 90 degrees, feet according to butt chest set to the left lower arm (elbow beneath shoulder) and corresponding to the top of the mat with left hand resting sitting on the hip. Press heels in a slurry, then lift left knee towards ceiling without altering the posture of the rest of your body. Then lower the knee and never lose heel alignment. It's one repetition. Do two sets that are 20 reps on each side.

Bowing sideboard

The best method for begin lying on the right side with legs bent to 90 degrees, heels aligned with butts, chest region set in the right lower arm (elbow beneath shoulder) that is parallel to the mat's top, with left hand resting to hip. Use lower arm press to raise hips until the body is in a straight lines from shoulders to knees. Do this for 30 seconds, after which you can lower them to start in a controlled manner and repeat the exercise the opposite side.

Book opening stretch

Instructions for step-by-step start lying on the right side, with your legs bent to 90 degrees, feet aligned with butts, hands tied behind heads, with elbows extending out to meet the face. While not moving your hips, rotate the left elbow, and then move your upper body to the reverse. Restart the exercise with control. This is one repetition. Perform 6 reps on either side.

Chest lift incline

Bit-by-bit guidelines for start lying down on your stomach with legs across the floor and also laying your temples on your hands, arms broad asleep on mat. Engage the middle section button to assist the lower back. Take your chest, shoulders as well as arms several steps off the ground using lower muscles of the back. Then, gradually increase the distance to start. It's one repetition. Perform two arrangements with 10 repetitions.

Bird Dog

The best method for begin is to sit on your feet with all fours, placing shoulder-width wrists and knees beneath hips. Straighten left arm ahead to increase height while you stretching the right leg until it reaches standing height. Make sure to hold it for a while, ensuring your shoulders and hips are aligned with the ground. Begin by lowering back. This is one repetition. Do 10 reps for both sides.

Jackass kick

The best method for begin is to sit on all fours, with your arms under shoulders, and knees underneath the hips. Bring stomach button back up, then into the back to link by abdominal muscles. With the leg in a twisted position at 90 degrees, extend the left leg until the thigh aligns with flooring without curving lower back. Begin to lower down. It's one repetition. Perform two sets of fifteen reps on each side.

Bowing board

Most effective way to start is on your feet with hands behind shoulders and knees underneath hips. The shoulders should be pushed forward above the wrists, and lower hips towards bottom until the body forms a single straight line from the top of the head to knees. Tailbones are folded inward, expanding between shoulder bones and collarbones while drawing the your paunch button towards the your spine. Do this for 30-60 seconds.

Full board

The best method for begin is to sit on your feet with hands behind shoulders, knees beneath hips. Toes are tucked. Then, push shoulders forward over wrists, and raise knees from mat in order to form a long line that extends from the crown of the heads to the heels. The tailbone is folded slightly, expanding through collarbones and the shoulder bones. Then, pull stomach button to the side towards the spine. Keep it for 30-60 seconds.

Squat

Instructions for: Begin standing feet separated by hips in addition to being equally. Pivot between the hips, pull butts back, then sink down until the you have thighs that are equal to the the floor. The chest should be slightly advancé and straighten arms in front of you to help balance your body. Maintain knees in line with your adjacent toes. Push into your heels and stay on the heels using your glutes to gain strength. This is a single repetition. Do two sets of 15 reps.

Hip pivot and jump

Most effective way to start is by putting yourself in a lurch using the left leg extended in front of your body, toes folded, impact point high and the right leg extending forward with knee level and foot bow, arms secured before your chest.

Chapter 16: The 5 Amazing & Great Exercise Moves To Put Right Into Your Weekly Activities (For Fibromyalgia Symptoms)

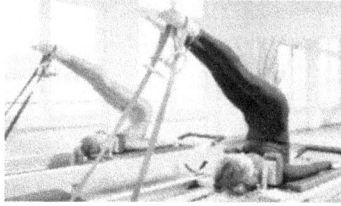

The best exercise options are in the following order:

Pelvic Clocks

It's a great way to gain confidence in your body. Learn how to release your abs and pelvis whilst remaining in a position to keep the rest of your body in a relaxed state.

1. Relax on your back and place your knees bent with your feet firmly on the ground. Be sure that your legs are in the same position in width, and your hips apart. Relax your neck and shoulders. Cut the shoulders to your ears. Put your hands onto your hips.

2. Imagine a clock that is at the hipbones' level twelve o'clock lies at your bellybutton. six o'clock is your pelvic bone in addition to the 9 and 3 o'clocks on your hipbones.

3. Work your abs to the max and also tilt your pelvis slightly to raise your back. Your pelvic bone (6 hours) ought to be more elevated. Keep your very chest portion loose.

4. Use your abdominal muscles to move your pelvis to ensure that the hip that is at 3 o'clock will be lower. Continue to move non-stop and shifting your pelvis around 6 o'clock, and the next time you lift your hip, it's 9 o'clock.

5. Rehash in the opposite method. Rehash several times.

Twisted Knee Fall Outs

This exercise works lower abs, the oblique and internal thighs along with the quadriceps. It is also excellent for pelvic floor exercises.

1. Lay on the floor while keeping your knees bent, with your feet at a level in addition to keeping your spine straight and with a slight bent.

2. The shoulder bones should be dragged down on your back. Keep the shoulders separated from the ear to flatten the capulae (shoulder bone skeletons).

3. Breathe in, pull the belly button in, then engage your abdominal muscles.

4. When you breathe your breath out and let your left knee slowly open up and move to the side. Do not lift your hip bones. Notice a slight stretch along your thigh's inner thighs.

5. When you breathe the air, gently move your knee and bring it back into focus.

6. Rehash with the opposite leg.

7. Rehash to eliminate 5 repetitions for each leg. Zero into keeping your abs in place.

Span

The activity that targets your hindquarters and lower back can help build strong muscles for your glutes and legs. This can cause back pain as well as stress.

1. Relax on your back, while your legs are bent and your feet are level with the flooring.

2. Relax and raise your legs off the floor until you are well-organized. Push your glutes to the side and then draw into your middle. Do 1 rep to the top of your development.

3. Be sure to keep your shoulders flat on the ground and don't extend your back too far at the top. Do not curve over your shoulders.

4. Return to the beginning and repeat the 5 steps several times.

Heel Slides

This exercise focuses on the abs in the lower part and should be performed in socks, on a smooth area.

1. Lay on the floor by knees bent. your feet at a level and an unbending spine and with a slight bending.

2. Make sure you draw your shoulder bones to towards your back and in order for scapulae support.

3. Breathe in, pull your belly button and then align your abs.

4. The next time you breath out slowly fix your knee while shifting your heels along the flooring. Keep your spine pelvis still.

5. When you breathe and out, move your knee slowly returning to the starting place.

6. Rehash with the opposite leg.

7. Rehash five redundancies for each leg. Concentrate on stability by the pelvis and also using the lower abdominals to help move the leg.

Chapter 17: Some Important Questios As Well As Answers About Pilates

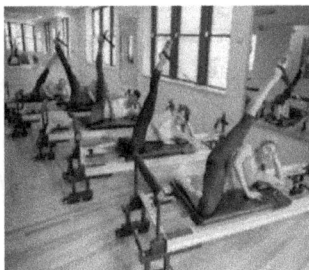

What's the main difference between Pilates as well as yoga?

Both modalities as well the different ways they are taught incorporate breathing adjustments to the body and a relaxing long. A lot of classes incorporate elements from the two, but Pilates and yoga aren't all alike.

In general, Pilates is more dynamic than yoga. That's the main reason why people are attracted to it. Studies have revealed. It is my opinion that people view it as slow-moving or just to sit and think. The body can play a role in the same reason, based on your class, but I was astonished by the amount of testing it did for my body completely novel method.

In yoga, you stand in static positions and In Pilates you maintain a steady rate. Your breathing techniques also vary depending on the post-exercise radiance increases. Following yoga, you have to slowly move to your daily routine.

Do you think that you could lose weight by doing Pilates?

It's not often known for falling numbers on the scale when you're in a hurry, like concentrated training for energy, but these short and repetitive exercises stimulate your heart, so it will consume some calories.

These small movements also pull muscles upwards from your top to bottom. The muscles will be strengthened, stretched and tonify. Feeling a little tingly the next day indicates that the muscles have recovered and that your new normal is functioning.

Pilates is done near the floor. It is possible to be seated, adjusted to your back, or lying on your back while you are getting into shape each turns.

What are the benefits of Pilates?

Pilates routines are often recommended to reduce the strain on joints, muscle stiffness as well as back discomfort as well as to aid in preventing injuries. If you are suffering from or are suffering from any of the above but you are not sure, consult your physician prior to starting any exercises.

They are easy to learn and master regardless of ability or age. If you want to improve your performance and add hand weights and extend your stretches to increase your consumption. Are you unable to cope with injury? Be relaxed about it. Pilates is flexible by design.

As we see improvements on a the world at large the last few years, it appears that this time, the income will have a significant impact on public perceptions through the vast economic business sectors.

These benefits extend beyond your time on the mat or machine Studies have revealed

Finding ways to keep your inner center even in the simplest of tasks such as putting on clothes, distributing food or having kids can help you over the long run, as studies demonstrate. Your mind will be more balanced. There will be less issues when you get older along with losing muscles. It will be possible to maintain flexibility and adaptability and also continue to enjoy the movement.

How can I get things going through Pilates?

It's best to get an experienced teacher who will take you through the steps with the proper structure. there is a possibility that you will learn by you will be taught one-on-one or as part of a group class.

www.ingramcontent.com/pod-product-compliance
Lightning Source LLC
Chambersburg PA
CBHW060222030426
42335CB00014B/1312